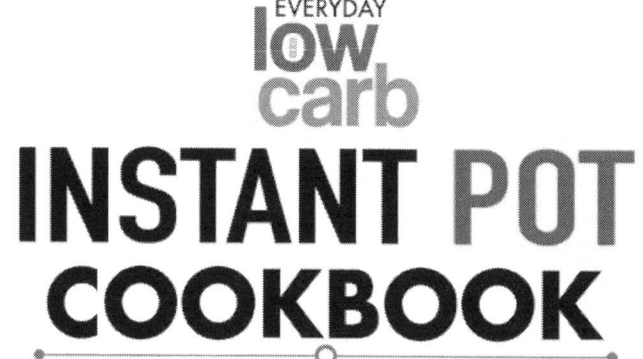

INSTANT POT COOKBOOK

30 DELICIOUS, *LOW CARB ELECTRIC PRESSURE COOKER RECIPES* FOR WEIGHT LOSS

Copyright © 2016 Linda Stevens
All Right Reserved.

Published by The Fruitful Mind LTD.

Disclaimer

The information in this book is not to be used as medical advice. The recipes should be used in combination with guidance from your physician. Please consult your physician before beginning any diet. It is especially important for those with diabetes, and those on medications to consult with their physician before making changes to their diet.

All rights reserved. No part of this publication or the information in it may be quoted from or reproduced in any form by means such as printing, scanning, photocopying or otherwise without prior written permission of the copyright holder.

Disclaimer and Terms of Use: Effort has been made to ensure that the information in this book is accurate and complete, however, the author and the publisher do not warrant the accuracy of the information, text and graphics contained within the book due to the rapidly changing nature of science, research, known and unknown facts and internet. The Author and the publisher do not hold any responsibility for errors, omissions or contrary interpretation of the subject matter herein. This book is presented solely for motivational and informational purposes only.

Table of Contents

INTRODUCTION 5
SOUPS AND STEWS 11
    GARLIC BEEF STEW 12
    CHILI BLANCO 14
    SMOKED SCALLOP CHOWDER 16
    TUSCAN CHICKEN STEW 18
    SPEEDY POSOLE 20
CHICKEN DISHES 23
    LEMONGRASS CHICKEN 24
    HONEY BALSAMIC CHICKEN 26
    RUSTIC CHICKEN AND ACORN SQUASH 28
    JERK CHICKEN 30
    ISLAND CHICKEN 32
    KIEV STYLE CHICKEN 34
    OLD WORLD OLIVE AND ARTICHOKE CHICKEN 36
    TANGERINE CHICKEN 38
    CHICKEN CACCIATORE 40
BEEF DISHES 43
    ITALIAN STYLE ROAST TIPS 44
    ROSEMARY BEEF AND MUSHROOMS 46
    HORSERADISH ROAST WITH PEARL ONIONS 48
    GARLIC BEEF AND BROCCOLI 50
    NO CRUST PIZZA CASSEROLE 52
    GREEN CURRIED BEEF STEAK 54
PORK DISHES 57
    TENDERLOIN FLORENTINE 58
    SAGE STUFFED PORK CHOPS 60
    PINEAPPLE AND LIME FAJITAS 62
    SPICY PEANUT PORK 64

Maple Dijon Tenderloin 66
Sunshine Coast Pork 68

VEGETARIAN DISHES 71
No" Mac" and Cheese 72
Wild Mushroom Ragu 74
Vegetarian Curry 76
Ready in a Minute Squash Casserole 78
Gingery Vegetables 80
Quicker Than Take Out Hot Pot 82

CONCLUSION 84

Introduction

The stove top pressure cooker has been around for ages. Chances are that somewhere along the line, you have known someone who has used one, and along with their knowledge of the pressure cooker come stories of disaster and exploding dinners dripping from the ceiling. While stove top pressure cookers still do exist, a new generation of pressure cookers have entered the scene; the electric pressure cooker. The electric pressure cooker is an amazing cooking device, capable of cooking an incredibly wide variety of delicious dishes, including those that fit into your low carb lifestyle.

Low carb cooking is incredibly quick and easy when using an electric pressure cooker because the device was created to cook the very foods that make up your healthy lifestyle. Meats cook up juicy and tender, while vegetables cook to the perfect texture to highlight their flavors in just a matter of minutes. For many of us, it can become a struggle to prepare healthy homemade meals on a regular basis. The time involved is just too much of a strain on our already hectic schedules. With an electric pressure cooker, the task of making a healthy, wholesome, low carb meal ends up taking only minutes, rather than hours. Soon, more and more of your meals will be eaten at home, made from ingredients that you have chosen that are healthy and at their peak of ripeness. What could be better than nourishing your body with these healthy, low carb foods on a daily basis?

One of the biggest healthy advantages to pressure cooking is the fact that food is cooked using simple liquids, such as water or broth, with tastes and textures that normally would require an abundance of fats and oils in other styles of cooking. Pressure cooking is also very budget friendly, which is a major benefit, especially for lifestyles that can sometimes be more costly to the budget, such as low carb diets. Even the least expensive cuts of meat can be dressed with spices and browned to a nice golden color before undergoing the pressure cooking process, with the result being one of the most rich and tender pieces of meat that has ever melted in your mouth.

But what about all of the bad things that you have heard about pressure cookers? You have probably heard that pressure cookers are dangerous, they explode, meats end up tough, etc. The truth is that yes, sometimes these things have happened, but they resulted from less than careful use. Modern electric pressure cookers are equipped with safety devices that indicate the amount of pressure, along with measure to ensure that the device does not open during cooking. There are multiple speeds of reducing the pressure, along with capabilities to perform cooking techniques beyond that of simple pressure cooking. Great culinary achievements can be crafted in your electric pressure cooker, with nothing more than a respect for the device and an understanding of how to use it.

Advice and Tips for Successful Cooking with Your Electric Pressure Cooker

Understand the pressure settings and PSI for your electric pressure cooker. While most electric pressure cookers will come with similar features, some models will still be more basic, while others boast more bells and whistles. One area that you will need to understand your piece of equipment and how it translates to successful recipes is in the pressure settings. Some electric pressure cookers will come with a low and high pressure setting, while others will have a low, medium and high. In general, the lowest pressure setting will cook at approximately 220°f with a pressure of 3psi (pounds per square inch). The medium pressure setting will cook at approximately 235°F with a pressure of 10psi. The high pressure setting will cook at approximately 250°F with a pressure of 13-15psi. This is where reading your instruction manual will greatly affect the results of your cooking. Use the suggested pressure settings for certain foods according to what your manual says, even if it is different from the recommended settings outlined in these recipes. These recipes have been formulated with general instructions, which are meant to serve a wide variety of pressure cookers and be adjusted as needed for best results. If your manual states to cook a certain food on medium or low pressure, but the recipe in this book states high pressure, you should choose to follow the advice of the manufacturer of your pressure cooker.

Know the difference between quick and natural release. Your pressure cooker will likely come with two steam and pressure release settings; a quick release and a natural release. The descriptions of these is intuitive in the fact that the quick release means that the pressure is quickly released from the pressure cooker, while the natural release takes much longer, but is a gentler, more natural process. In most cases, you will want to use the quick release when adding additional ingredients part way through cooking. The natural release can be used at the end of cooking. The natural release slightly extends the cooking time and leads to a more tender and fully cooked final product.

Make sure that you have the proper amount of food and liquid in your pressure cooker for it to work properly. The recipes in this book have been formulated to fit a 4-6L size pressure cooker. Since pressure cookers can vary so much in size and capacity, you may have to adjust the ingredients to suit your equipment. In general, you do not want to fill your pressure any more than two thirds of the way full with total contents. Overfilling will result in proper pressure not building up and your food simply won't cook. Your pressure cooker also needs liquid to build the steam and pressure. Most pressure cookers will work fine with at least one cup of liquid, however you should follow the instructions in your model's manual for advice on the proper amount of liquid to add.

Timing will take some practice, but eventually it will become intuitive. In the beginning, you might need to spend some time experimenting with your electric pressure cooker and what settings to cook on and for how long. Even if you are a pro at cooking with a stovetop pressure cooker, or have used a different electric pressure cooker in the past, you will likely experience a period of adjustment. Just remember that as you experiment it is best to start low and build pressure and cooking times as needed. You can always go back and cook something a little bit more if it isn't completely cooked.

Make sure your pressure cooker is at the proper pressure before you start counting cooking times. Let say you are cooking something with a recommended ten minutes cooking time at high pressure. Those ten minutes only start once the pressure cooker indicates that it has achieved the chosen pressure level. If you start counting before pressure is achieved, your food will be undercooked.

Brown your meat a little before building up pressure. Most electric pressure cookers come with a brown or sauté setting. Use this to lightly brown your meats before adding the liquid and other ingredients. This will add a richness and additional flavor and texture to your dishes.

Cut your ingredients evenly. Evenly sized pieces are going to cook evenly at one setting. If you cut up your meat into many different sized pieces you are likely to end up with some that are overcooked and some that are undercooked. The same applies to vegetables and other ingredients. Also, when adding multiple ingredients, consider density against size. If you are adding cubed potatoes and broccoli to a dish and want to add them at the same time and want them to reach appropriate doneness at the same time, then you will need to accommodate for this by cutting the denser potatoes into smaller cubes, while using less dense larger pieces of broccoli.

Some things won't work no matter how hard you try. It is near impossible to get a sauce to reduce in a pressure cooker; there just isn't the opportunity for evaporation. Baking requires dry heat, so if you attempt to cook anything with dough, like pie, you will just end up with a soggy mess. Never add dairy early in the cooking, as it will curdle under the pressure. Dairy should only be added during the last couple of minutes, or after the pressure cooking has taken place. The same is true for many herbs, which will lose much of their flavor if added too soon.

Don't be afraid to experiment. Once you are comfortable with your electric pressure cooker, you will begin to realize that the options for culinary delights are endless, especially options to suit your low carb lifestyle.

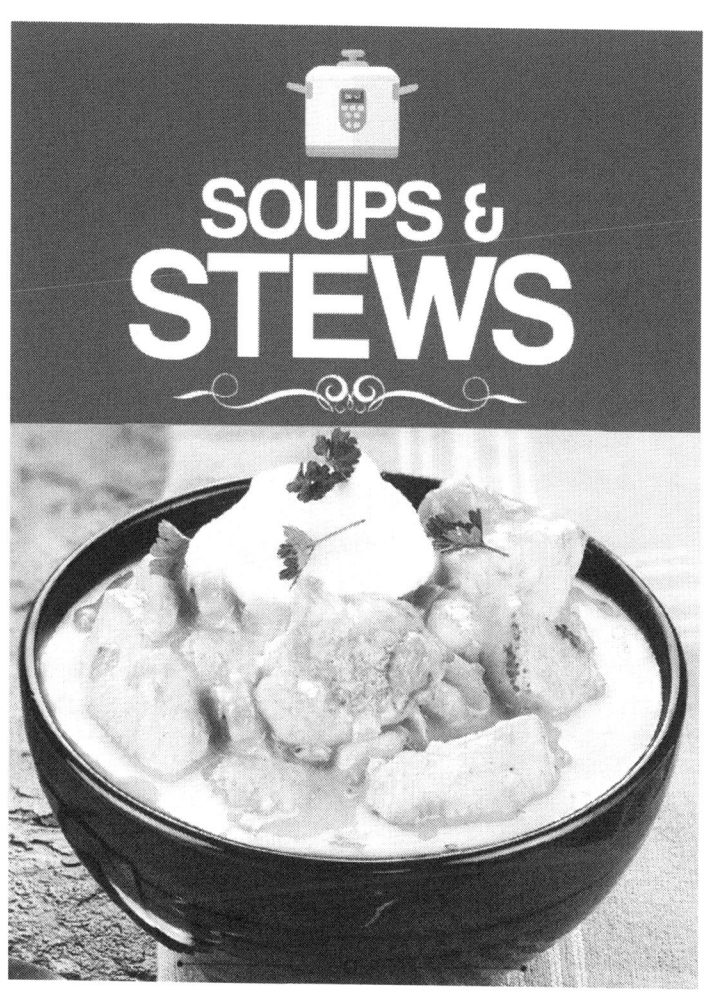

Garlic Beef Stew

Serves: 8
Nutritional Information: Calories 215, Fat 6.5g, Protein 20.3g, Net Carbohydrates 14.1g

Ingredients:
1 lb beef stew meat
1 teaspoon salt
1 teaspoon black pepper
1 tablespoon cornstarch
2 tablespoons olive oil
6 whole cloves garlic
1 ½ cup pearl onions
2 cups carrots, sliced thick
2 cups sweet potatoes, cubed into 1 inch pieces
3 cups beef stock, or enough to completely cover the ingredients
2 tablespoons soy sauce
2 tablespoons Worcestershire sauce
1 tablespoon honey
1 tablespoon fresh thyme
1 sprig fresh rosemary

Directions:
Set up and prepare your electric pressure cooker according to manufacturer's instructions. Turn your pressure cooker on the "brown" or "sauté" setting.

Combine the salt, pepper and cornstarch and lightly dredge the stew meat through the mixture. Add the olive oil and garlic cloves to the pressure cooker and lightly brown the meat for 2-3 minutes.

In a bowl combine the beef stock, soy sauce, Worcestershire sauce, honey, thyme and rosemary. Add the mixture to the browned stew meat.

Close and seal the pressure cooker and set the pressure to high. Cook for 10-12 minutes. Using the quick release, release the steam and add the pearl onions, carrots and sweet potatoes.

Bring the steam back up to high and cook for an additional 7-10 minutes, or until meat is cooked through and vegetables are tender.

Chili Blanco

Serves: 6
Nutritional Information: Calories 213, Fat 6g, Protein 23g, Net Carbohydrates 12.8g

Ingredients:
1 lb chicken, cut into cubes
1 teaspoon salt
1 teaspoon black pepper
3 cloves garlic, crushed and minced
1 ½ cup cauliflower florets
2 tablespoons olive oil
3 cups chicken stock
1 cup yellow onion, sliced
1 cup poblano pepper, cut into small cubes
2 cups canned white kidney beans, rinsed and drained
½ cup roasted tomatillo salsa, or salsa verde
1 teaspoon chili powder
2 teaspoons cumin
¼ cup fresh cilantro, chopped
Lime wedges for garnish
Sliced scallions for garnish

Directions:
Set up and prepare your electric pressure cooker according to manufacturer's instructions. Turn your pressure cooker on the "brown" or "sauté" setting.

Season the chicken with salt and black pepper. Add the olive oil to the pressure and then the chicken and garlic. Sauté for 2-3 minutes.

Add the cauliflower and the chicken stock. Close and seal the pressure cooker and set the pressure to high. Cook for 10-12 minutes.

Using the quick release, release the steam.

Add in the onion, poblano pepper, white kidney beans, roasted tomatillo salsa or salsa verde, chili powder, cumin and cilantro.

Cover and bring the pressure back up to high. Cook for an additional 5-7 minutes, or until chicken is cooked through.

Stir well to distribute the cauliflower, which should be soft enough to add a creamy consistency to the chili. Garnish with scallions and lime wedges for serving.

Smoked Scallop Chowder

Serves: 6
Nutritional Information: Calories 222, Fat 7g, Protein 19g, Net Carbohydrates 14g

Ingredients:
½ lb bacon, diced
2 cloves garlic, crushed and minced
1 tablespoon olive oil
½ cup shallots, diced
1 cup celery, chopped
1 cup carrots, chopped
2 ½ cups butternut squash, cubed into 1 inch pieces
3 cups fish stock, or enough to completely cover ingredients
½ cup dry white wine
1 teaspoon liquid smoke, add more or less to taste
1 tablespoon fresh thyme
1 teaspoon salt
1 teaspoon white pepper
1 lb scallops
1 ½ cup whole milk
Sliced scallions for garnish

Directions:
Set up and prepare your electric pressure cooker according to manufacturer's instructions. Turn your pressure cooker on the "brown" or "sauté" setting.

Add the bacon, garlic and olive oil. Sauté until the bacon is browned, approximately 3-4 minutes.

Add the shallots, celery, carrots, butternut squash, fish stock, dry white wine and liquid smoke.

Cover and seal the pressure cooker and set the pressure to high. Cook for 5 minutes.
Using the quick release, release the steam.

Add in the thyme, salt, pepper and scallops. Bring the pressure back up to high and cook for 3-5 minutes, or until scallops are cooked through.

Release the steam and add the milk. Stir well and let set while it cools slightly.

Garnish with sliced scallions.

Tuscan Chicken Stew

Serves: 6
Nutritional Information: Calories 210, Fat 8g, Protein 22g, Net Carbohydrates 11.6g

Ingredients:
1 lb chicken, cut into 1 inch cubes
3 cloves garlic, crushed and minced
2 tablespoons olive oil
2 15 ounce cans crushed tomatoes with liquid
2 cups chicken stock
2 ears fresh corn, cut into quarters
2 cups portabella mushrooms, halved or quartered
1 cup green bell pepper, chopped
¼ cup fresh parsley, chopped
¼ cup fresh basil, chopped
1 sprig fresh rosemary
1 tablespoon fresh thyme
1 teaspoon paprika
1 teaspoon salt
1 teaspoon black pepper

Directions:
Set up and prepare your electric pressure cooker according to manufacturer's instructions. Turn your pressure cooker on the "brown" or "sauté" setting.

Add the olive oil, chicken and garlic to the pressure cooker and brown for 2-3 minutes.

Add the crushed tomatoes with liquid and chicken stock.

Cover and seal the pressure cooker. Set the pressure to high and cook for 15 minutes. Using the quick release, release the steam.

Add in the corn, mushrooms, bell pepper, parsley, basil, rosemary, thyme, paprika, salt and black pepper.

Cover and bring the pressure back up to high. Cook for an additional 5-7 minutes, or until chicken is cooked through and vegetables are tender.

Speedy Posole

Serves: 4
Nutritional Information: Calories 385, Fat 18g, Protein 37g, Net Carbohydrates 13g

Ingredients:
1 lb pork, cubed
1 tablespoon olive oil
2 cloves garlic, crushed and minced
2 cups chicken stock
2 cups green enchilada sauce
1 cup yellow onion, diced
1 cup poblano pepper, diced
1 ½ cup white hominy
½ cup fresh cilantro, chopped
1 teaspoon cumin
1 teaspoon onion powder
1 teaspoon salt
1 teaspoon black pepper
Sliced radish for garnish
Lime wedges for garnish

Directions:
Set up and prepare your electric pressure cooker according to manufacturer's instructions. Turn your pressure cooker on the "brown" or "sauté" setting.

Add the olive oil, pork and garlic to the pressure cooker. Sauté for 2-3 minutes.

Add the chicken stock and enchilada sauce.

Cover and seal the pressure cooker. Set the pressure to high and cook for 10-12 minutes. Using the quick release, release the steam.

Add in the onion, poblano pepper, hominy, cilantro, cumin, onion powder, salt and black pepper.

Cover and bring the pressure back up to high. Cook for an additional 3-5 minutes or until pork is cooked through. Serve garnished with radish and lime.

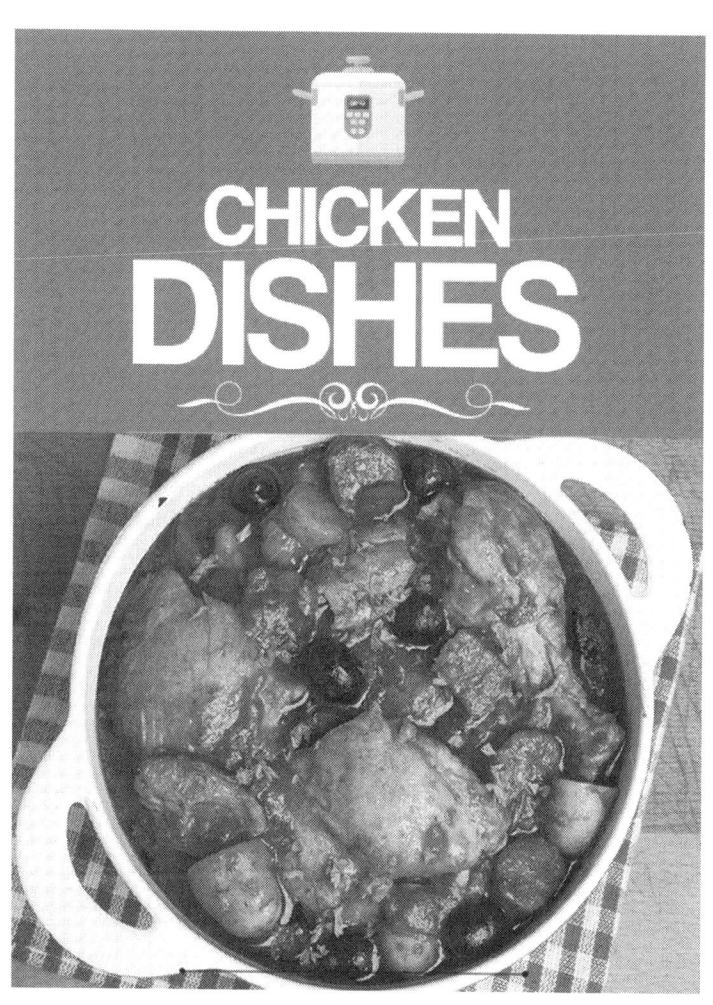

Lemongrass Chicken

Serves: 4
Nutritional Information: Calories 212, Fat 7g, Protein 29g, Net Carbohydrates 6g

Ingredients:
1lb bone in chicken pieces
1 tablespoon olive oil
2 cloves garlic, crushed and minced
1 cup yellow onion, sliced
1 cup chicken stock
½ cup soy sauce
1 tablespoon fresh grated ginger
1 tablespoon fresh lemongrass, chopped
1 tablespoon lime juice
1 teaspoon black pepper

Directions:
Set up and prepare your electric pressure cooker according to manufacturer's instructions.

Turn your pressure cooker on the "brown" or "sauté" setting.

Add the olive oil, chicken and garlic to the pressure cooker and brown the meat for 2-3 minutes.

Add the onion, chicken stock, soy sauce, ginger, lemongrass, lime juice and black pepper.

Cover and seal the pressure cooker. Set the pressure to high and cook for 15-20 minutes or until chicken is cooked through.

Honey Balsamic Chicken

Serves: 4
Nutritional Information: Calories 239, Fat 7g, Protein 30g, Net Carbohydrates 13g

Ingredients:
1 lb bone in chicken pieces
1 tablespoon olive oil
2 cloves garlic, crushed and minced
1 cup red onion, sliced
1 cup chicken stock
¼ cup balsamic vinegar
1 tablespoon honey
1 sprig fresh rosemary
3 cups asparagus spears, chopped
¼ cup fresh basil, chopped
1 teaspoon salt
1 teaspoon coarse ground black pepper

Directions:
Set up and prepare your electric pressure cooker according to manufacturer's instructions.

Turn your pressure cooker on the "brown" or "sauté" setting. Add the olive oil, chicken and garlic to the pressure cooker and brown for 2-3 minutes.

Combine the chicken stock, balsamic vinegar, and honey. Add to the pressure cooker, along with the red onion and rosemary.

Cover and seal the pressure cooker. Set the pressure to high and cook for 15 minutes. Using the quick release, release the steam.

Add in the asparagus, basil, salt and black pepper.

Cover and bring the pressure back up to high. Cook for an additional 5 minutes, or until chicken is cooked through.

Rustic Chicken and Acorn Squash

Serves: 4
Nutritional Information: Calories 240, Fat 7g, Protein 29g, Net Carbohydrates 11g

Ingredients:
1 lb bone in chicken pieces
1 teaspoon ground sage
1 tablespoon olive oil
2 cloves garlic, crushed and minced
1 cup chicken stock
1 cup yellow onion, sliced
2 cups acorn squash, cubed
2 cups portabella mushrooms, halved
1 teaspoon oregano
1 teaspoon salt
1 teaspoon black pepper

Directions:
Set up and prepare your electric pressure cooker according to manufacturer's instructions. Turn your pressure cooker on the "brown" or "sauté" setting.

Season the chicken with the ground sage. Add the olive oil and chicken to the pressure cooker and brown for 2-3 minutes.

Add the garlic and chicken stock. Cover and seal the pressure cooker. Set to high and cook for 15 minutes.

Using the quick release, release the steam. Add the onion, acorn squash, mushrooms, oregano, salt and black pepper.

Cover and bring the pressure back up to high. Cook an additional 5 minutes, or until chicken is cooked through.

Jerk Chicken

Serves: 4
Nutritional Information: Calories 271, Fat 7g, Protein 28g, Net Carbohydrates 14g

Ingredients:
1 lb bone in chicken pieces
½ teaspoon cinnamon
½ teaspoon nutmeg
½ teaspoon allspice
1 teaspoon black pepper
1 tablespoon olive oil
4 cloves garlic, crushed and minced
1 cup yellow onion, sliced
1 tablespoon jalapeno pepper, diced
1 cup chicken stock
½ cup orange juice
1 tablespoon honey
2 teaspoons crushed red pepper flakes
1 cup red bell pepper, cubed
1 cup fresh pineapple chunks
1 cup acorn squash, cubed

Directions:
Set up and prepare your electric pressure cooker according to manufacturer's instructions. Turn your pressure cooker on the "brown" or "sauté" setting.

Season the chicken with cinnamon, nutmeg, allspice and black pepper.

Add the olive oil and garlic to the pressure cooker along with the chicken. Brown the chicken for 2-3 minutes.

Combine the chicken stock, orange juice, honey and crushed red pepper flakes. Mix well and add to the pressure cooker, along with the onion and jalapeno pepper.

Cover and seal the pressure cooker. Set the pressure to high and cook for 15 minutes. Using the quick release, release the steam.

Add in the red bell pepper, fresh pineapple and acorn squash.

Cover and bring the pressure back up to high. Cook an additional 5 minutes, or until the chicken is cooked through.

Island Chicken

Serves: 6
Nutritional Information: Calories 255, Fat 11g, Protein 23g, Net Carbohydrates 13g

Ingredients:
1 lb boneless, skinless chicken breasts
1 teaspoon salt
1 teaspoon black pepper
1 tablespoon olive oil
1 clove garlic, crushed and minced
1 tablespoon fresh grated ginger
1 cup chicken stock
¼ cup Worcestershire sauce
2 tablespoons orange juice
1 tablespoon lime juice
1 teaspoon allspice
1 teaspoon Serrano pepper, diced
3 cups sugar snap peas, trimmed
½ cup fresh pineapple chunks
½ cup peanuts, chopped

Directions:
Set up and prepare your electric pressure cooker according to manufacturer's instructions.

Turn your pressure cooker on the "brown" or "sauté" setting.

Season the chicken with salt and black pepper.

Add the olive oil to the pressure cooker, followed by the garlic, ginger and chicken.

Brown the chicken for 2-3 minutes.

In a bowl combine the chicken stock. Worcestershire sauce, orange juice, lime juice, allspice and Serrano pepper. Mix well and add to the pressure cooker.

Cover and seal the pressure cooker. Set the pressure to high and cook for 15 minutes.

Using the quick release, release the pressure.

Add in the sugar snap peas, pineapple chunks and peanuts.

Cover and bring the pressure back up to high. Cook an additional 5 minutes, or until chicken is cooked through.

Kiev Style Chicken

Serves: 4
Nutritional Information: Calories 412, Fat 27g, Protein 30g, Net Carbohydrates 7g

Ingredients:
1 lb boneless, skinless chicken breasts
1 teaspoon salt
1 teaspoon black pepper
½ cup butter
3 cloves garlic, crushed and minced
1 cup red onion, sliced
1 cup chicken stock
¼ cup dry white wine
4 cups broccoli florets
½ cup fresh parsley, chopped
¼ cup fresh tarragon

Directions:
Set up and prepare your electric pressure cooker according to manufacturer's instructions. Turn your pressure cooker on the "brown" or "sauté" setting.

Season the chicken with salt and black pepper. Add the butter and garlic to the pressure cooker and let the butter melt before adding the chicken.

Brown the chicken in the butter for 2-3 minutes. Add in the onion, chicken stock and dry white wine.

Cover and seal the pressure cooker. Set the pressure to high and cook for 15 minutes. Using the quick release, release the steam.

Add the broccoli, parsley and tarragon. Cover and bring the pressure back up to high.

Cook and additional 3-5 minutes, or until chicken is cooked through.

Old World Olive and Artichoke Chicken

Serves: 4
Nutritional Information: Calories 346, Fat 14g, Protein 30g, Net Carbohydrates 15g

Ingredients:
4 boneless, skinless chicken breasts
1 teaspoon salt
1 teaspoon black pepper
1 tablespoon olive oil
3 cloves garlic, crushed and minced
1 cup chicken stock
½ cup dry white wine
2 cups white mushrooms, quartered
2 cups tomatoes, chopped
1 cup artichoke hearts, quartered
¼ cup fresh parsley, chopped
1 teaspoon oregano
1 teaspoon thyme
½ cup green olives, sliced

Directions:
Set up and prepare your electric pressure cooker according to manufacturer's instructions. Turn your pressure cooker on the "brown" or "sauté" setting.

Season the chicken with salt and black pepper. Add the olive oil, garlic and chicken to the pressure cooker and brown the chicken for 2-3 minutes.

Add the chicken stock and dry white wine. Cover and seal the pressure cooker. Set the pressure to high and cook for 15 minutes.

Using the quick release, release the steam. Add the mushrooms, tomatoes, artichoke hearts, parsley, oregano, thyme and green olives.

Cover and bring the pressure back up to high. Cook an additional 3-5 minutes, or until the chicken is cooked through.

Tangerine Chicken

Serves: 4
Nutritional Information: Calories 249, Fat 7g, Protein 29g, Net Carbohydrates 11g

Ingredients:
1 lb boneless, skinless chicken breast
1 teaspoon salt
1 teaspoon black pepper
1 tablespoon olive oil
1 cup chicken stock
¼ cup tangerine or orange juice
1 tablespoon lime juice
1 tablespoon tangerine zest
1 teaspoon Serrano pepper, diced
1 tablespoon paprika
2 cups broccoli florets
2 cups carrots, sliced thick

Directions:
Set up and prepare your electric pressure cooker according to manufacturer's instructions. Turn your pressure cooker on the "brown" or "sauté" setting.

Season the chicken with salt and black pepper. Add the olive oil and chicken to the pressure cooker and brown the chicken for 2-3 minutes.

In a bowl combine the chicken stock, orange juice, lime juice, tangerine zest, Serrano pepper and paprika. Mix well and add to the pressure cooker.

Cover and seal the pressure cooker. Set the pressure to high and cook for 15 minutes. Using the quick release, release the steam.

Add the broccoli and carrots. Cover and bring the pressure back to high. Cook an additional 3-5 minutes, or until chicken is cooked through.

Chicken Cacciatore

Serves: 4
Nutritional Information: Calories 237, Fat 7g, Protein 29g, Net Carbohydrates 8g

Ingredients:
1 lb bone in chicken pieces
1 teaspoon salt
1 teaspoon black pepper
1 tablespoon olive oil
4 cloves garlic, crushed and minced
1 28 oz can crushed tomatoes, including liquid
1 cup chicken stock
¼ cup dry red wine
1 cup green bell pepper, cubed
2 cups portabella mushrooms, halved
¼ cup fresh basil
¼ cup fresh oregano

Directions:
Set up and prepare your electric pressure cooker according to manufacturer's instructions. Turn your pressure cooker on the "brown" or "sauté" setting.

Season the chicken with salt and black pepper. Add the olive oil along with the garlic and chicken to the pressure cooker. Brown the chicken for 2-3 minutes.

Add the tomatoes, including the liquid, chicken stock and dry red wine to the pressure cooker.

Cover and seal the pressure cooker. Set the pressure to high and cook for 15 minutes.

Using the quick release, release the steam. Add the green bell pepper, portabella mushrooms, basil and oregano.

Cover and bring the pressure back to high. Cook for 3-5 minutes, or until the chicken is cooked through.

BEEF DISHES

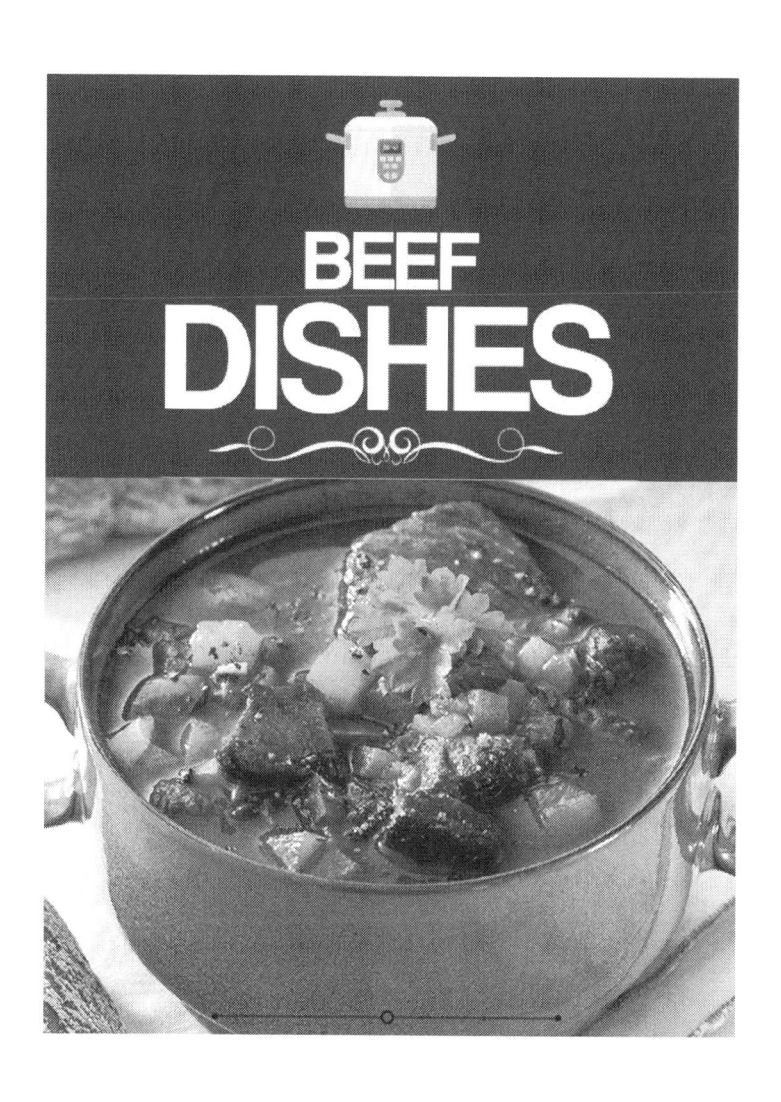

Italian Style Roast Tips

Serves: 4
Nutritional Information: Calories 301, Fat 13g, Protein 38g, Net Carbohydrates 5g

Ingredients:
1 lb sirloin beef tips
1 teaspoon salt
1 teaspoon black pepper
3 cloves garlic, crushed and minced
1 tablespoon olive oil
1 cup red onion, sliced
1 cup diced tomatoes
1 cup beef stock
2 tablespoons balsamic vinegar
6 cups fresh spinach
½ cup fresh basil, chopped
¼ cup fresh parsley, chopped
1 teaspoon oregano

Directions:
Set up and prepare your electric pressure cooker according to manufacturer's instructions. Turn your pressure cooker on the "brown" or "sauté" setting.

Season the beef tips with salt and black pepper. Add the olive oil and garlic to the pressure cooker and brown the meat for 2-3 minutes.

Add the remaining ingredients and stir. Cover and seal the pressure cooker. Set the pressure to high and cook for 15-17 minutes, or until beef tips reach desired doneness.

Rosemary Beef and Mushrooms

Serves: 4
Nutritional Information: Calories 344, Fat 13g, Protein 39g, Net Carbohydrates 11g

Ingredients:
1 lb beef stew meat
1 teaspoon salt
1`teaspoon coarse ground black pepper
2 teaspoons corn starch
2 cloves garlic, crushed and minced
1 tablespoon olive oil
½ cup beef stock
½ cup tomato juice
¼ cup dry red wine
1 sprig fresh rosemary
2 cups wild mushrooms, halved
1 cup red onion, sliced
4 cups fresh green beans, trimmed
1 teaspoon oregano
1 teaspoon onion powder

Directions:
Set up and prepare your electric pressure cooker according to manufacturer's instructions. Turn your pressure cooker on the "brown" or "sauté" setting.

In a bowl combine the salt, black pepper and corn starch. Lightly dredge the stew meat through the corn starch mixture.

Add the olive oil, garlic and stew meat to the pressure cooker. Brown the meat for 2-3 minutes.

Add the beef stock, tomato juice, dry red wine and rosemary to the pressure cooker.

Cover and seal the pressure cooker. Set the pressure to high and cook for 12 minutes.

Using the quick release, release the steam. Add in the mushrooms, onion, green beans, oregano and onion powder.

Cover and bring the pressure back to high. Cook an additional 3-5 minutes, or until meat has reached desired doneness.

Horseradish Roast with Pearl Onions

Serves: 6
Nutritional Information: Calories 534, Fat 34g, Protein 45g, Net Carbohydrates 5g

Ingredients:
2-3 lb beef roast (cut into smaller pieces, if needed to properly fit in your pressure cooker)
1 teaspoon salt
1 teaspoon coarse ground black pepper
1 tablespoon prepared horseradish
2 tablespoons olive oil
1 cup beef stock
¼ cup dry red wine
¼ cup Worcestershire sauce
4 cups fresh green beans, trimmed
1 cup pearl onions
1 teaspoon thyme
1 teaspoon oregano

Directions:
Set up and prepare your electric pressure cooker according to manufacturer's instructions. Turn your pressure cooker on the "brown" or "sauté" setting.

Season the roast with salt, black pepper and horseradish. Add the olive oil to the pressure cooker and brown the meat for 4-5 minutes.

Add the beef stock, dry red wine and Worcestershire sauce. Cover and seal the pressure cooker. Set the pressure to high and cook for 40 minutes.

Using the quick release, release the steam. Add the green beans, onions, thyme and oregano.

Cover and bring the pressure back to high. Cook an additional 3-5 minutes, or until meat has reached desired doneness.

Garlic Beef and Broccoli

Serves: 4
Nutritional Information: Calories 313, Fat 16g, Protein 37g, Net Carbohydrates 11g

Ingredients:
1 lb flank steak, cut into strips
1 teaspoon salt
1 teaspoon black pepper
1 tablespoon corn starch
4 cloves garlic, crushed and minced
2 tablespoons olive oil
½ cup beef stock
½ cup soy sauce
1 teaspoon sesame oil
1 tablespoon brown sugar
4 cups broccoli florets
1 cup yellow onion, diced
½ cup water chestnuts, chopped
Sliced scallions for garnish

Directions:
Set up and prepare your electric pressure cooker according to manufacturer's instructions. Turn your pressure cooker on the "brown" or "sauté" setting.

Combine the salt, black pepper and corn starch. Lightly dredge the steak through the corn starch mixture.

Add the olive oil, garlic and steak to the pressure cooker and brown the meat for 2-3 minutes.

In a bowl combine the beef stock, soy sauce, sesame oil and brown sugar. Mix well and add to the pressure cooker.

Cover and seal the pressure cooker. Set the pressure to high and cook for 12-15 minutes. Using the quick release, release the steam.

Add the broccoli, onion and water chestnuts. Cover and bring the pressure back to high. Cook and additional 3-5 minutes or until the meat is cooked to desired doneness.

No Crust Pizza Casserole

Serves: 4
Nutritional Information: Calories 452, Fat 30g, Protein 32g, Net Carbohydrate 9

Ingredients:
1 lb ground beef
3 cloves garlic, crushed and minced
2 cups diced canned tomatoes, with liquid
½ cup beef stock
1 teaspoon crushed red pepper flakes
1 cup white mushrooms, sliced
1 cup green bell pepper, diced
1 cup yellow onion, diced
2 cups fresh spinach
¼ cup fresh basil, chopped
1 teaspoon oregano
1 teaspoon salt
1 teaspoon black pepper
½ cup fresh mozzarella cheese
¼ cup fresh grated parmesan cheese

Directions:
Set up and prepare your electric pressure cooker according to manufacturer's instructions.

Add the ground beef, garlic, canned tomatoes with liquid, beef stock and crushed red pepper flakes to the pressure cooker.

Cover and seal the pressure cooker. Set the pressure to high and cook for 10 minutes. Using the quick release, release the steam.

Add in the mushrooms, green bell pepper, yellow onion, spinach, basil, oregano, salt and black pepper. Cover and bring the pressure back up to high.

Cook and additional 3-5 minutes, or until the meat is cooked through. Release the pressure and stir in the mozzarella and parmesan cheese. Allow the cheese to melt while the casserole cools.

Green Curried Beef Steak

Serves: 4
Nutritional Information: Calories 351, Fat 23g, Protein 26g, Net Carbohydrate 7g

Ingredients:
1 lb flank steak, cut into strips
1 teaspoon salt
1 teaspoon black pepper
2 cloves garlic, crushed and minced
1 tablespoon olive oil
1 cup beef stock
1 cup coconut milk
¼ cup soy sauce
1 tablespoon lime juice
1-2 teaspoons green curry paste
1 tablespoon fresh grated ginger
1 tablespoon fresh lemongrass, chopped
3 cups cabbage, sliced
1 cup carrots, grated

Directions:
Set up and prepare your electric pressure cooker according to manufacturer's instructions. Turn your pressure cooker on the "brown" or "sauté" setting.

Season the steak with salt and black pepper. Add the olive oil to the pressure cooker, along with the garlic and steak. Brown the meat for 2-3 minutes.

In a bowl combine the beef stock, coconut milk, soy sauce, lime juice, green curry paste, ginger and lemongrass. Mix well and add to the pressure cooker.

Cover and seal the pressure cooker. Set the pressure to high and cook for 12-15 minutes. Using the quick release, release the steam. Add the cabbage and carrots.

Cover and bring the pressure back up to high. Cook for an additional 2-3 minutes, or until meat has reached desired doneness.

PORK DISHES

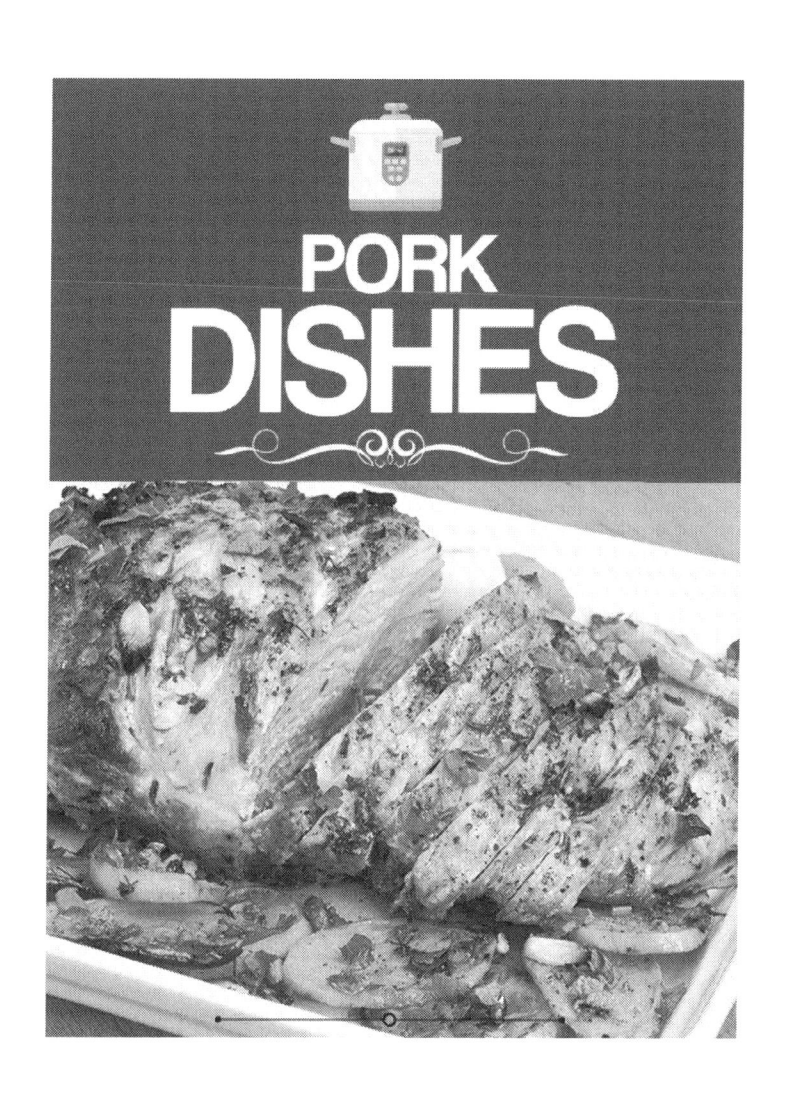

Tenderloin Florentine

Serves: 6
Nutritional Information: Calories 432, Fat 22g, Protein 48g, Net Carbohydrates 4g

Ingredients:
2-3 lb pork tenderloin, cut into smaller pieces, if necessary to accommodate your pressure cooker
1 teaspoon salt
1 teaspoon black pepper
2 cloves garlic, crushed and minced
1 tablespoon olive oil
1 cup chicken stock
1 teaspoon crushed red pepper flakes
½ cup dry white wine
6 cups fresh spinach
1 cup red onion, sliced
1 sprig fresh rosemary
½ cup heavy cream
½ cup fresh grated parmesan
Fresh parsley for garnish

Directions:
Set up and prepare your electric pressure cooker according to manufacturer's instructions. Turn your pressure cooker on the "brown" or "sauté" setting.

Season the pork tenderloin with salt and black pepper. Add the olive oil to the pressure cooker, along with the garlic and tenderloin.

Brown the meat for 3-5 minutes. Add the chicken stock and dry white wine.

Cover and seal the pressure cooker. Set the pressure to high and cook for 40 minutes.

Using the quick release, release the steam. Add the spinach, red onion, rosemary, heavy cream and parmesan.

Cover and bring the pressure back up to high. Cook for an additional 3-5 minutes, or until the meat is cooked through. Serve garnished with fresh parsley.

Sage Stuffed Pork Chops

Serves: 4
Nutritional Information: Calories 376, Fat 18g, Protein 36g, Net Carbohydrates 11g

Ingredients:
4 bone in pork chops
2 cups mushrooms, chopped
2 cups spinach, chopped
1 cup red onion, diced
2 teaspoons ground sage
¼ cup walnuts, chopped
1 teaspoon salt
1 teaspoon black pepper
1 teaspoon onion powder
1 tablespoon olive oil
1 cup chicken or vegetable stock
4 cups green beans, trimmed

Directions:
Set up and prepare your electric pressure cooker according to manufacturer's instructions. Turn your pressure cooker on the "brown" or "sauté" setting.

In a bowl combine the mushrooms, spinach, red onion, sage and walnuts. Mix well. Slice the pork chops along one side, going about two thirds of the way through the meat.

Stuff the mushroom mixture into the center of each pork chop. Season the outside of each pork chop with salt, black pepper and onion powder.

Place the olive oil in the pressure cooker, along with the pork chops and brown the meat for 2-3 minutes. Add the vegetable stock.

Cover and seal the pressure cooker. Set the pressure to high and cook for 25-30 minutes. Using the quick release, release the steam.

Add in the green beans. Cover and bring the pressure back up to high. Cook an additional 3-5 minutes, or until meat is cooked through.

Pineapple and Lime Fajitas

Serves: 4
Nutritional Information: Calories 313, Fat 13g, Protein 34g, Net Carbohydrates 11g

Ingredients:
1 lb pork, cut into strips
1 teaspoon salt
1 teaspoon black pepper
1 teaspoon chili powder
1 teaspoon cumin
1 teaspoon paprika
1 tablespoon olive oil
1 cup chicken or vegetable stock
1 tablespoon lime juice
1 cup red bell pepper, sliced
1 cup green bell pepper, sliced
1 cup yellow onion, sliced
1 cup fresh pineapple chunks, sliced
Large lettuce leaves for serving
Avocado, for garnish

Directions:
Set up and prepare your electric pressure cooker according to manufacturer's instructions. Turn your pressure cooker on the "brown" or "sauté" setting.

Season the pork with the salt, black pepper, chili powder, cumin and paprika. Add the olive oil, along with the pork to the pressure cooker. Brown the meat for 2-3 minutes.

Add the chicken or vegetable stock and lime juice. Cover and seal the pressure cooker. Set the pressure to high and cook for 12-15 minutes.

Using the quick release, release the steam. Add in the red bell pepper, green bell pepper, yellow onion and pineapple chunks.

Cover and bring the pressure back up to high. Cook for an additional 3-5 minutes, or until meat is cooked through. Serve in lettuce leaves, garnished with avocado.

Spicy Peanut Pork

Serves: 4
Nutritional Information: Calories 420, Fat 20g, Protein 40g, Net Carbohydrates 13g

Ingredients:
1 lb boneless pork, cubed
1 teaspoon salt
1 teaspoon black pepper
1 tablespoon olive oil
1 cup tomatoes, chopped
2 cups chicken or vegetable stock
¼ cup creamy peanut butter, no sugar added
1 tablespoon jalapeno pepper, diced
1 tablespoon fresh lemongrass
2 cloves garlic, crushed and minced
½ teaspoon cinnamon
1 teaspoon cumin
1 cup yellow onion, sliced
2 cups fresh green beans, trimmed
2 cups cabbage, sliced

Directions:
Set up and prepare your electric pressure cooker according to manufacturer's instructions. Turn your pressure cooker on the "brown" or "sauté" setting.

Season the pork with salt and black pepper. Add the olive oil along with the pork to the pressure cooker. Brown the meat for 2-3 minutes.

Add in the tomatoes, chicken stock, peanut butter, jalapeno pepper, lemongrass, garlic, cinnamon and cumin.

Cover and seal the pressure cooker. Set the pressure to high and cook for 12-15 minutes. Using the quick release, release the steam. Add in the onion, green beans and cabbage.

Cover and bring the pressure back up to high. Cook for an additional 3-5 minutes, or until meat is cooked through.

Maple Dijon Tenderloin

Serves: 6
Nutritional Information: Calories 361, Fat 14g, Protein 36g, Net Carbohydrates 10g

Ingredients:
2-3 lb pork tenderloin roast, cut into smaller pieces, if necessary to accommodate your pressure cooker
¼ lb peppered bacon, diced
1 tablespoon Dijon mustard
2 tablespoons maple syrup
2 cloves garlic, crushed and minced
1 teaspoon salt
1 teaspoon black pepper
2 tablespoons olive oil
1 ½ cup chicken or vegetable stock
1 cup yellow onion, sliced
2 cups Brussels sprouts, halved
1 tablespoon fresh dill
1 tablespoon fresh chives, chopped

Directions:
Set up and prepare your electric pressure cooker according to manufacturer's instructions. Turn your pressure cooker on the "brown" or "sauté" setting.

In a bowl combine the Dijon mustard, maple syrup, garlic, salt and black pepper. Mix well and spread the mixture over the pork.

Add the olive oil and bacon to the pressure cooker. Cook the bacon for 2 minutes before adding the tenderloin. Brown the tenderloin for 2-3 minutes.

Add in the chicken or vegetable stock. Cover and seal the pressure cooker. Set the pressure to high and cook for 25-30 minutes. Using the quick release, release the steam.

Add in the Brussels sprouts, onion, dill and chives. Cover and bring the pressure back to high. Cook and additional 5 minutes, or until the meat is cooked through.

Sunshine Coast Pork

Serves: 4
Nutritional Information: Calories 344, Fat 13g, Protein 37g, Net Carbohydrates 13g

Ingredients:
1 lb boneless pork, cubed
1 teaspoon salt
1 teaspoon black pepper
1 teaspoon coriander
2 cloves garlic, crushed and minced
1 tablespoon jalapeno pepper, diced
1 tablespoon olive oil
1 cup chicken or vegetable stock
½ cup orange juice
¼ cup lime juice
1 tablespoon honey
1 teaspoon lemon zest
1 cup leeks, sliced
2 cups broccoli florets

Directions:
Set up and prepare your electric pressure cooker according to manufacturer's instructions. Turn your pressure cooker on the "brown" or "sauté" setting.

Season the pork with salt, black pepper and coriander. Add the olive oil to the pressure cooker along with the pork, garlic and jalapeno pepper. Brown the meat for 2-3 minutes.

In a bowl combine the chicken stock, orange juice, lime juice, honey and lemon zest. Mix well and add to the pressure cooker.

Cover and seal the pressure cooker. Cook for 12-15 minutes. Using the quick release, release the steam.

Add in the leeks and broccoli. Cover and bring the pressure back up to high. Cook an additional 3-5 minutes, or until the meat is cooked through.

VEGETARIAN DISHES

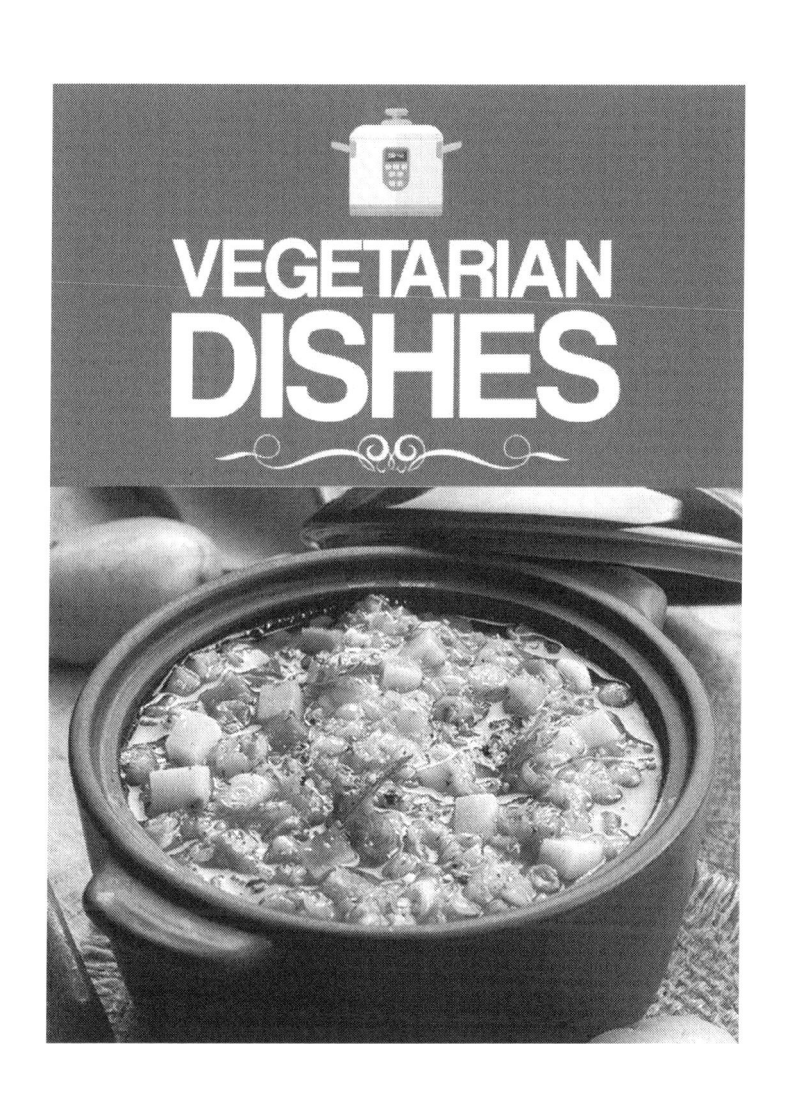

No" Mac" and Cheese

Serves: 6
Nutritional Information: Calories 450, Fat 32g, Protein 24g, Net Carbohydrates 12g

Ingredients:
1 large head cauliflower, cut into small florets
1 cup yellow onion, diced
1 cup red bell pepper, diced
1 cup vegetable stock
1 teaspoon salt
1 teaspoon black pepper
1 cup extra sharp cheddar cheese, grated
1 cup swiss cheese, grated
½ cup goat cheese
½ cup heavy cream
1 teaspoon Dijon mustard
1 teaspoon nutmeg
1 tablespoon fresh chives

Directions:
Set up and prepare your electric pressure cooker according to manufacturer's instructions.

Add the cauliflower, onion, red bell pepper, vegetable stock, salt and black pepper to the pressure cooker.

Cover and seal the pressure cooker. Set the pressure to high and cook for 5-6 minutes.

In a bowl combine the cheddar cheese, Swiss cheese, goat cheese, heavy cream, Dijon mustard, nutmeg and chives.

Release the pressure and remove the lid. While the contents are still hot, stir in the cheese mixture. Let set while the dish cools slightly before serving.

Wild Mushroom Ragu

Serves: 4
Nutritional Information: Calories 251, Fat 18g, Protein 11g, Net Carbohydrates 10g

Ingredients:
6 cups wild mushrooms or other mushroom variety, halved
1 cup leeks, sliced
2 cloves garlic, crushed and minced
2 cups tomato, chopped
1 tablespoon olive oil
4 cups spinach, torn
1 ½ cup vegetable stock
1 teaspoon nutmeg
1 teaspoon salt
1 teaspoon coarse ground black pepper
½ cup walnuts, chopped
½ cup goat cheese, crumbled

Directions:
Set up and prepare your electric pressure cooker according to manufacturer's instructions.

Add all of the ingredients, except for the goat cheese to the pressure cooker.

Cover and seal the pressure cooker. Set the pressure to high and cook for 3-4 minutes.

Release the steam and remove the lid.

Stir in the goat cheese and let melt while the dish cools slightly before serving.

Vegetarian Curry

Serves: 6
Nutritional Information: Calories 138, Fat 5g, Protein 6g, Net Carbohydrates 14g

Ingredients:
2 cup carrots, cut thick
½ cup celery, chopped
1 cup yellow onion, sliced
4 cups cauliflower florets
2 cups green beans, trimmed
1 cup tomatoes, chopped
4 cups fresh spinach, torn
2 cups vegetable stock
½ cup coconut milk
1 ½ tablespoon curry powder
1 tablespoon honey
1 tablespoon fresh lemongrass, chopped
1 tablespoon fresh grated ginger
2 teaspoons crushed red pepper flakes
1 teaspoon salt
1 teaspoon black pepper
Fresh basil for garnish

Directions:
Set up and prepare your electric pressure cooker according to manufacturer's instructions.

Add the sweet potatoes, carrots, celery, onion, cauliflower, green beans, tomatoes and spinach to the pressure cooker.

In a bowl combine the vegetable stock, coconut milk, curry, honey, lemongrass, ginger, red pepper flakes, salt and black pepper. Mix well and add to the pressure cooker.

Cover and seal the pressure cooker. Set the pressure to high and cook for 3-4 minutes.

Slowly release the steam and let cool slightly before serving.

Ready in a Minute Squash Casserole

Serves: 4
Nutritional Information: Calories 304, Fat 25g, Protein 11g, Net Carbohydrate 9g

Ingredients:
4 cups yellow summer squash, sliced
½ cup red onion, chopped
1 cup tomatoes, chopped
2 cups cremini mushrooms, quartered
1 cup vegetable stock
1 teaspoon salt
1 teaspoon black pepper
1 teaspoon oregano
½ teaspoon nutmeg
½ cup walnuts, chopped
½ cup heavy cream
½ cup fresh grated parmesan cheese

Directions:
Set up and prepare your electric pressure cooker according to manufacturer's instructions.

Add all of the ingredients, except for the parmesan cheese to the pressure cooker.

Cover and seal the pressure cooker. Set the pressure to high and cook for 3-4 minutes.

Release the steam and stir in the parmesan cheese before serving.

Gingery Vegetables

Serves: 6
Nutritional Information: Calories 94, Fat 2g, Protein 3g, Net Carbohydrates 12g

Ingredients:
2 cups broccoli florets
2 cups snow peas, trimmed
2 cups green beans, trimmed
2 cups carrots, sliced
1 cup yellow onion, sliced
1 cup water chestnuts
1 cup vegetable stock
¼ cup ponzu or soy sauce
2 teaspoons sesame oil
¼ cup orange juice
2 cloves garlic, crushed and minced
1 tablespoon fresh grated ginger
1 teaspoon salt
1 teaspoon black pepper

Directions:
Set up and prepare your electric pressure cooker according to manufacturer's instructions.

Add the broccoli, snow peas, green beans, carrots, yellow onion and water chestnuts to the pressure cooker.

In a bowl combine the vegetable stock, ponzu or soy sauce, sesame oil, orange juice, garlic, ginger, salt and black pepper. Mix well and add to the pressure cooker.

Cover and seal the pressure cooker. Set the pressure to high and cook for 3-4 minutes or until vegetables are crisp tender.

Quicker Than Take Out Hot Pot

Serves: 2-4
Nutritional Information: Calories 142, Fat 3g, Protein 9g, Net Carbohydrates 13g

Ingredients:
3 cups bok choy, sliced
1 cup oyster mushrooms, chopped
1 cup shitake mushrooms, chopped
2 cups edamame, shelled
1 cup yellow onion, sliced
1 cup carrot, sliced thin
2 cup zucchini, julienned
4 cups vegetable stock
2 tablespoons ponzu or soy sauce
1 tablespoon rice vinegar
2 teaspoons sesame oil
1 tablespoon crushed red pepper flakes
2 star anise pods
1 teaspoon cardamom pods
½ teaspoon salt
1 teaspoon black pepper
Sliced scallions for garnish

Directions:
Set up and prepare your electric pressure cooker according to manufacturer's instructions.

In a bowl combine the vegetable stock, ponzu or soy sauce, rice vinegar, sesame oil, crushed red pepper, star anise, cardamom, salt and black pepper. Mix well and add to the pressure cooker.

Add the remaining ingredients, except for the scallions to the pressure cooker.

Cover and seal the pressure cooker. Set the Pressure to high and cook for 3-5 minutes. Garnish with fresh scallions before serving.

Conclusion

We all want to be healthy, and if you have made the commitment to living a life where your dietary choices align with those desires, then you know that sometimes life can get in the way of making those decisions easy. We are all busy, and on top of it, many of us are accustomed to a lifestyle of instant gratification. Why spend the time preparing and waiting for a meal to cook, when there is another option that will be ready in just a matter of minutes? Unfortunately, most of the time it is our health that suffers in those situations. But these obstacles can be overcome, one such way being the use of an electric pressure cooker to help you create easy, new and exciting low carb dishes to enjoy every day.

Low carb eating does not need to be a challenge, and you do not have to stick with the same old dishes time and time again. With an electric pressure cooker, you can add new life and vitality to your daily meals with dishes that can literally be prepared in minutes and be on the table in no time at all. What I hope that you have gained from this book is the inspiration to overcome your fear or intimidation of pressure cookers and to realize the limitless potential of deliciousness that awaits.

Made in the USA
Lexington, KY
19 March 2019